Free playlists are available by
following Shannon Yrizarry
on Spotify.

Namaste.

Contents:

1. Inversions
2. Backbends & Forward Folds
3. Hip Opening
4. Well Rounded Class
5. Mandala Class
6. Level 2 Class
7. Peak Pose Class
8. Open Level Class
9. Spine Strengthening Class
10. Twisting Class
Bonus Restorative Class

Inversions Class
Theme: Take a new perspective (How can you look at things differently to fuel your passion/goals?)

Intro: Feet up the wall, embryo, puppy pose, squat reach w/ heels down, Fordward fold, Standing Splits, Forward fold, Down dog

Section A: Forward Fold, ½ way lift, Forward Fold, Tadasana, one legged Tadasana, Warrior 3, standing splits, Forward fold (Do Right side then Left side)

Section B: Down Dog, Warrior 1, Humble Warrior, Forward fold w/ clasped hands, tadasana w/ clasped hands, W3 w/ clasped hands, exalted warrior, chaturanga to handstand jump-back (Right/Left)

Core: Down dog to dolphin one arm at a time, Down dog, Plank, knee to Right/nose/left through and flip to falling star

Inversions: Headstand, Forearm stand, tripod, candlestick, wheel x 3

Standing: Prasarita, Dancers w/ reverse hand grip, down dog, Titibasana (firefly)

Hips: Seated ½ pigeon, butterfly, runners lunge, seated grab big toe pull back, ½ lotus w/ bent legs and fold forward, Lotus lift!

Shoulders: standing bring each arm flat on wall on at a time first perpendicular to wall then at a 45 degree angle, Cow with hands at shoulder height on Wall, thread the needle

Cool Down: Dragon fly (straddle forward fold), supine twist, savasana

Inversions help heart health, strengthen the diaphragm to improve lung function during tough activities, ease back pain by taking pressure off disks, and reduce stress by decreasing the body's fight or flight response.

Be Humble.

Backbends and Forward Folds Class (Spinal Elasticity and Hamstrings)
Theme: Tell Yourself You Deserve Love, (What are you telling yourself that doesn't serve you?)
Props: 2 blankets, 2 blocks

Intro: Bolster under lower back lie flat, embryo, table top (grab opposite foot and arch back), Down Dog, Dolphin (lift one leg bend knee towards head), Down Dog, walk hands forward to Forward Fold

Section A: Low Lunge, Low Crescent Lunge (circle arms to backbend), ½ pigeon pull back heel in, crescent lunge (circle arms to back bend), tadasana, arms up w/ steeple grip bend right/left and back, Forward Fold (do right side then left side)

Section B: Forward Fold, Chair Pose, Warrior 3 steeple grip, ½ moon, reverse half moon, ½ moon grab foot and arch back, runners lunge, back foot in, Extended Side Angle w/ bind, high crescent lunge (eagle arms arch back)

Core: 10 yogi pushups (chaturanga w/ breath), side plank (grab top foot and back bend), crow hold 5 seconds to jump back x3

Standing: Dancer's w/ strap on ankle and between big toe like a flip flop (2 arm grab over head), Reverse big toe pose, padanhastasana, padangustasana, prasarita, interlace hands on 2nd prasarita

Inversions: Candlestick (with 2 blankets under shoulders), Plow Pose (long hold), Headstand (long hold), Headstand leg lifts, Childs Pose, Standing Splits to handstand

Backbends: bow pose, Wheel or bridge (lift one leg) x3, camel, vipparita

Splits: Frog, ½ hanuman, full hanuman asana

Forward Folds: ½ dragonfly, ½ lotus with forward fold, marichyasana A, marichyasana B, dragonfly, kurmasana (long hold), dandasana (bolster under legs)

Cool down: 2 blocks under shoulders in T position (one between shoulder blades, one under head), ½ sleeping pigeon, straight leg supine twist and reverse reclined big toe pose w/ schwastica, hug knees small circles, savasana

YOU DESERVE LOVE

Accept yourself as you are. Otherwise you will never see opportunity. You will not feel free to move toward it. You will feel you are not deserving. -Maxwell Maltz

Be Consistent.

Hip Opening Class
Props: One Block, Three blankets

Intro: Standing Steeple Grip Bend Right and Left, Seated Fan Legs Twist spine, Plank bring one leg to floor near hip and turn on side of feet dropping hips then lift hips reaching arm over head

Section A: Tadasana, Interlace hands to Forward Fold, one legged tadasana w/ hand clasp, warrior 3 w/ clasp, giva squat hands in prayer, squat and curl (do Right side then left)

Section B: Forward Fold, float to Down Dog, rockstar, Low Lunge, Extended Side Anlge arm swings, gate pose back/forward, goddess squat, up to toes, Warrior 2 facing back of room, humble warrior, tadasana. (do right and left sides twice)

Core: Forward Fold lift heel bring leg to side/forward, stretch pose 20 seconds, boat pose (row your boat)

Inversions: Handstand or handstand prep to straddle

Extra strength: Malasana, side crow, padahastasana, Low Lunge, crescent lunge, crescent twist, prayer twist, Forward Fold (Right side then left side)

Standing: Prasarita, figure 4, tree w/ bind to toe stand balance, Standing Splits

Backbends: Camel, dropbacks, wheel to forearm stand straight legs (viparita)

Hips: seated pigeon, ½ lord of the fishes, cow face, fire log, ½ sleeping pigeon

Shoulders: seated arm across chest, pull elbow above head, lock fingers behind bac

Cool down: Halasana (plow pose optional w/ blankets under shoulders)

Savasana

May We Exude Loving Kindness

"There Must Be Consistency in Direction."-W. Edwards Demming

Relax.

Well Rounded Class
Transformation: What can you transform?
**Makes Class 1 ½ Hr

Section A: Samastiti, Tadasana, Forward Fold, ½ Way Lift, Chaturanga, Down Dog (5 breaths), Forward Fold, ½ way Lift, Tadasana (x5)

Section B: Samastiti, Chair, Forward Fold, ½ Way Lift, Chaturanga, Down Dog, Warrior 1, Chaturanga, Forward Fold, ½ Way Lift, Tadasana, Samastiti (x5)

****Extra Core:** Plank lift one leg and arm, reverse plank, side plank

Inversions: Handstands on Wall

****Extra Inversion:** Headstand (hold 10 breaths)

Standing Poses: Warrior 2 (hold for 5 breaths), Extended Side Angle (hold for 5 breaths), Reverse Warrior (hold for 5 breaths), Chaturanga, Down Dog, Forward Fold, ½ Way Lift, Tadasana, (Other Side)

****Extra Standing Poses:** Dancer's (Hold 5 breaths), Eagle (Hold 5 breaths), Standing Pigeon (Hold 5 breaths), Triangle (Hold 5 breaths), Prasarita (Hold 5 breaths)

Backbends: Wheel (hold 5 breaths) x3

Arm Balance: Crow (hold 5 breaths)

Hip Openers: Butterfly (against wall), Runner's Lunge, ½ Sleeping Pigeon, ½ Lotus

Splits: Right/Left/Straddle

****Shoulders:** Cow w/ Hands on wall, shoulder's on wall standing one arm out right/left and at a 45 degree angle, thread the needle, roll over shoulder, 2 blocks stacked under elbows, lie on two blocks in a T

Cool Down: Plow

****Extra Cool Down:** ½ Lord of the fishes, Rabbit, Supine Twist

Savasana

You find freedom inside, no where else. In the heart of every human being is that one space which is free, which is filled with peace, and which is full of love. -Prem Rewatt

Be Colorful.

Mandala Class (Do something different for a new perspective)
Theme: Have fun
Props: 2 blocks, 1 Strap, 1 Blanket

Intro: Sufi Grind, Cat/Cow, Gate Pose, Puppy, Down Dog, Wild Thing, Down Dog, Float to Forward Fold

Section A: Chair, Forward Fold, Low Lunge, Extended Side Angle w/ Bind, Runners Lunge, Back Leg In, Plank, Side Plank to Tree, Down Dog (Right/Left side x2)

MANDALA Section B: Samastiti, Prasarita, One Shoulder then the other, Warrior 1 to back of room, Warrior 3, one legged tadasana, Big Toe (Right/Left side x 2)

Core: Pizza crunches (Flat body V-ups), Superman, Table top one leg out to side, plank lift one leg and opposite arm

Arm Balances: Runner's Lunge to shoulder under for Hurdler's Pose

Strength Building: Mountain Pose (arch back), Forward Fold, ½ way lift, Chaturanga, Down dog, one leg up, low lunge, high crescent lunge (eagle arms arch back), Warrior 2, Triangle, Warrior 2, Reverse Warrior, Chaturanga, Side Plank, Down Dog, Forward Fold, Chair, Prayer Twist, Gorilla (Right/Left side)

Splits: Crescent Moon, ½ Hanuman Asana, Righ/Left Splits (with blocks), Middle Splits (with blocks) Straddle on back

Inversions: Headstands (leg lifts), Donkey Kick ups, Standing Split Kick Ups

Backbends: Cobra, Cobra w/ Bent Legs, Walk hands down Wall, Wheel (x5)

Shoulders: Cow with hands on Wall at shoulder height, Elbows on Blocks walk knees back like puppy pose, thread the needle, wrist stretches

Forward Fold's: Sleeping Pigeon, Firelog, ½ Dragonfly w/ backwards knee, Straddle, Dandasana

Cooling: Suptapadangustasana w/ Strap (both sides go right and left), Plow, Sivasana on stomach

When the body is active, the mind can be free. -Shannon Yrizarry

Have Fun.

Level 2 Class
Theme: Expand Yourself

Intro: Swing Arms, Down Dog (5 breaths), Rag-doll, Low lunge, Forward Fold, Low Lunge, Plank, Down Dog

Section A: Forward Fold, ½ way Lift, Forward Fold, Samastiti, Mountain, Arch Back, Mountain, Forward Fold, ½ way Lift, Plank, Side Plank (both sides), Down Dog (x3)

Section B: Samastiti, Mountain, Arch, Mountain, Forward Fold, Chair, Prayer Twist, High Crescent Lunge, Crescent Twist, Arms Up, Humble Warrior, Stay Clasped, Warrior 3, Standing Splits, Warrior 2, Reverse Warrior, Extended Side Angle (Bind) (Right/Left side x3)

Standing: Padangustasana (5 breaths), Padanhastasana (5 breaths), Pyramid (5 breaths), Trianngle, Big Toe to Dancer's, Feathered Peacock, Standing Pigeon

Arm Balances: Crow, Figure 8, Firefly, peacock in Lotus

Inversions: Handstands, Forearm stands

Backbends: Locust, Cobra, Wheel (5 breaths x 5)

Core: Side Plank, On Back Alternate lowering Legs then Both Legs, Mountain Climbers, Forearm Plank Up/Downs

Hips: Splits, Seated Pigeon, ½ Sleeping Pigeon

Shoulders: Wall Stretches, Block stretches, prasarita (grab opposite leg and twist)

Forward Folds: Standing Forward Fold, Hands through, prasarita, happy baby, ½ Dragonfly, straddle

Cool Down: Plow, firelog, fish, rabbit, supine twist, savasana

Hold Space For Others.

Peak Pose Class: One Legged Flying Pigeon (Eka Pada Galavasana)
Props: 2 blocks

Warm Up: Swing Arms Side To Side, Down Dog, One legged Dog pose, Table Top, Thread the Needle, Plank, Forearm Plank, Dolphin, Down Dog, Forward Fold

Section A: Samastiti, Mountain, Arch back, Mountain, Forward fold, Malasana, Forward Fold, ½ Lift, Plank, Side Plank, Down Dog, Forward Fold (x3)

Section B: Samastiti, Mountain, Arch back, Mountain, Forward fold, step one leg back, crescent lunge, crescent twist, Extended Side Angle, reverse Extended Side Angle, runners, pull back foot in, low crescent, down-dog, (otherside)

Standing Poses: Warrior 2, Warrior 3, Half-moon, reverse half-moon, tree pose to toe pose, pyramid, big toe pose to dancers (otherside), standing forward fold with hands clasped, standing pigeon,

Core: Boat Pose, Reverse Plank, On back lower one leg at a time then both

Arm Balances: Crow Pose, One Legged Flying Pigeon

Back Bends: Camel, Cobra, Wheel x 5 (5 breaths each)

Inversions: Handstands (10 donkey kicks, then from standing splits) or Headstands (hold 20 seconds, bring legs up and down)

Forward Folds: ½ Dragon fly, Straddle, Seated figure four, Happy Baby, Plow, Seated forward fold, Lotus

Cool Down: Shoulder against the wall standing perpedicular to floor and at a 45 degree angle, elbows on two blocks, blocks under shoulders in a T (one under shoulder blades one under head), supine twist, savasana

Don't seek, don't search, don't ask, don't knock, don't demand-relax. If you relax, it comes, if you relax, it is there. If you relax, you start vibrating with it. -OSHO

Live From Your Heart.

Open Level Class

Intro: Swing Arms, Down Dog, One Legged Dog, Rag Doll, Samastiti

Section A: Mountain, Arch Back, Mountain, Forward Fold, ½ way Lift, Roll Back Plow, Forward Fold, ½ way Lift, Forward Fold, Samastiti (x3)

Section B: Mountain, Arch Back, Mountain, Forward Fold, Chair, Prayer Twist, Crescent Twist, Crescent Lunge w/ Arch Back, Crescent Moon Pose, Arch Back, Back heel In, ½ Hanuman, Forward Fold, Standing Splits, Warrior 2, Humble Warrior, Warrior 3, One Legged Tadasana (Right/Left side x3)

Core: Plank to forearm plank, Side Plank, On back R/L both, Reverse Plank, Rock n' Roll, boat pose x 5

Arm Balances: Crow, Child's Pose, Plank, Side Plank to Tree or Hanuman Asana,

Inversions: Headstand (lift lower legs), Donkey Kick up to Handstand, Standing Splits to Handstand,

Standing: Padangustasana, Forward Fold with hands clasped, Standing Pigeon, Big Toe Pose, Dancers, Pyramid, Triangle, Tree bound to forward fold to balancing toe stand, prasarita (grab toes, hands on ground, hands clasped)

Hip Openers: Seated ½ Pigeon, ½ Sleeping Pigeon, Firelog, lie on back straddle, runner's lunge

Back Bends: Locust, Cobra, Bow Pose, Legs Bent Cobra, Bridge, Wheel (x3)

Shoulder Openers: lie on 2 blocks, roll over shoulder, shoulders on wall, cow on wall, Shoulders on blocks, Dolphin, wrist stretches, toe stretches

Forward Folds: Straddle, ½ dragon fly, dandasana, marichyasana A, seated twists

Cool Down: Fish Pose, Rabbit, Plow, Supine, Happy Baby, Legs up the wall for Sivasana

Svadhaya is a yogic term referring to how we treat ourselves. It means being close to oneself, through meditation and self-exploration. It refers to knowing more about oneself intentionally. This helps us give up self-destructive tendencies. It teaches us to be centered and non-reactive.

Eat Healthy.

Spine Strengthening Class
Theme: An attitude of Trust to get you to your destination

Warm up: Standing Arms Swings, Seal pose, cat cow, Down dog, Forward Fold, Rag-doll, tadasana

Section A: Samastiti, Tadasana (arch back), Forward fold, ½ way lift, Forward fold, Chaturanga, Down Dog, Forward Fold (x3)

Section B: Tadasana, Forward fold, ½ way lift, Chair, Forward Fold, one leg lifts to wild thing, Low lunge, Warrior 1, Chaturanga, Down Dog, Forward Fold (Right/Left x3)

Core: Sit on knees interlace hands behind head lean right/left, side plank crunches, forward fold lift heel side forward front to toe stand without heel touching ground, table top

Strength Building: Down dog, high crescent lunge, arch back, crescent moon, back heel in, high crescent lunge twist, reverse warrior, chaturanga, Down dog, forward fold, prayer twist, forward fold (right side, left side)

Standing: Dancer's pose, Padanhastasana,

Hip Stretches: Mermaid, ½ sleeping pigeon, wild thing

Backbends: Flying locust, bow pose, bridge pose, wheel pose, camel, king pigeon (kapotasana)

Cool down: Shoulder stand, plow, fish pose, danurasana (5 breaths), savasana

They say think twice before you jump. I say jump first then think as much as you want. -OSHO

Show Compassion.

Twisting Class (Detox)
Theme: 2nd Chakra Balancing enhances our relationships, balances emotions and release guilt and resentment leaving room for creativity

Warm Up: Down dog, scorpion, high plank, knee to right shoulder, knee to nose, knee to left shoulder, knees touch toes together twist, butterfly

Section A: Forward fold, ½ Lift, Tadasana palms together, samastiti, tadasana palms together, forward fold, prayer twist, forward fold (right side/left side)

Section B: samastiti, Tadasana palms together, forward fold, ½ way lift, Forward fold, handstand, chair pose, forward fold, ½ way lift, chaturanga, down dog, low lunge, warrior 1, warrior 2, extended side angle, low lunge, chaturanga, down dog, forward fold (right side/left side x2)

Core: Hold plank on forearms, knee to shoulder and then alternate dropping knees, rest on side glute and pedal legs and arms, boat pose

Strengthening: Low lunge, high crescent lunge to twist, lizard pose, gorilla pose (right side/left side)

Hip Stretches: Samastiti, Tadasana, Triangle pose, feathered bird of paradise

Standing: Eagle pose, Dancer's pose, revolved standing big toe pose

Backbends: Half frog pose (cobra pulling heel to thigh)

Cool Down: Candlestick, Plow, ½ sleeping pigeon, seated ½ lord of the fishes, cow face pose, happy baby, supine twist with legs crossed and knees close to chest, savasana

Trust You Are Taken Care Of.

Bonus Restorative Class

(2 mins) Big Toe Pose

(5 mins each side) ½ Dragon Fly

(5 minutes) Full Dragon Fly

(4 minutes) 2 blocks in a T under shoulders lying down

(2 minute) Elbows on 2 blocks

(2 minutes on each side) Thread the Needle

(2 minutes on each side) roll over shoulder

(3 minutes) Reclined Supta Badha Konasana (with strap and blocks)

(2 minutes) Plum Line Pose

(4 minutes) Butterfly (folding forward)

(4 mins on each side) ½ sleeping pigeon

(2 mins) Supported bridge

(3 mins on each side) Supine Twist

(10 mins) Sivasana

Contact:

Shannon Yrizarry
syrizarry@gmail.com